PART 2

HOW TO DEAL

WITH

HEALTH CRISIS

Tips for long life

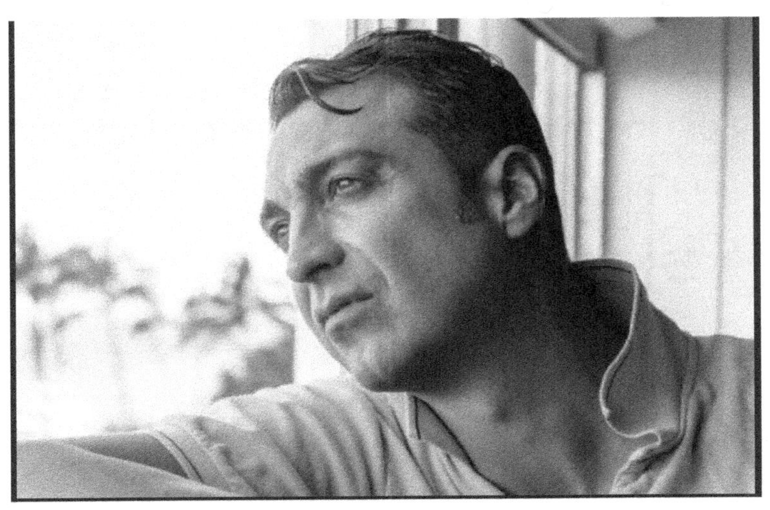

TABLE OF CONTENTS

Introduction

Once upon a time, there was a young woman named Emily who was diagnosed with a chronic illness. She felt lost and overwhelmed, unsure of how to cope with the challenges that lay ahead. As days turned into weeks and months, Emily's health deteriorated, and she found herself spending more and more time confined to her bed.

One rainy afternoon, while browsing through her bookshelf, Emily stumbled upon an old, dusty book titled "HOW TO DEAL WITH HEALTH CRISIS" Intrigued, she began to read, immersing herself in the stories and wisdom contained within its pages. The book spoke of the transformative power of literature, how words could soothe the soul and heal the body.

As Emily delved deeper into the book, she felt a sense of hope stirring within her. She started to incorporate the book's teachings into her daily routine, reciting affirmations and passages that resonated with her. Slowly but surely, she began to notice a change in herself. She felt stronger, more resilient, as if the words she read were infusing her with a newfound sense of purpose and determination.

With each passing day, Emily's health improved. She no longer felt as though she was merely surviving; she was thriving. Her journey was far from easy, but she faced each obstacle head-on, drawing strength from the words that had once seemed so distant and intangible.

Eventually, Emily emerged from her health crisis stronger than ever before. She credited her recovery not only to medical treatment but also to the healing power of the book that had guided her through the darkest days of her illness. And as she closed the final chapter of "The Healing Power of Words," she knew that she would carry its lessons with her for the rest of her life.

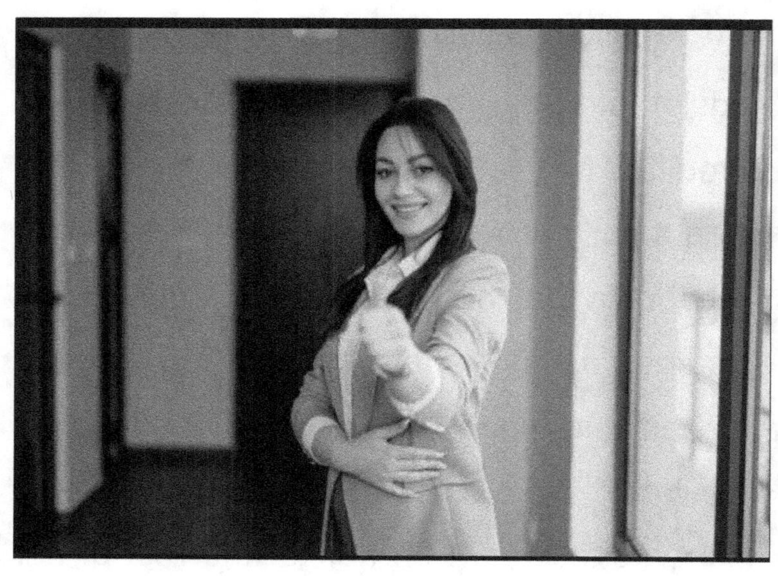

CHAPTER 1 : Long Term Planning and Management

Introduction:

In times of health crises, such as pandemics or large-scale disease outbreaks, long-term planning and management are crucial for effective response and recovery. While immediate actions are necessary to address the urgent needs, it's equally important to develop strategies that can mitigate future risks and build resilience within healthcare systems and communities. This comprehensive guide explores the key aspects of long-term planning and management in health crises, focusing on strategies to prepare for, respond to, and recover from such events.

Understanding Long-Term Planning in Health Crisis:

1. Risk Assessment and Preparedness:

- Conducting comprehensive risk assessments to identify potential health threats and vulnerabilities.

- Developing preparedness plans that outline strategies for early detection, rapid response, and resource allocation.

2. Infrastructure and Capacity Building:

- Investing in robust healthcare infrastructure, including hospitals, laboratories, and healthcare facilities, to enhance capacity during emergencies.

- Strengthening healthcare workforce capacity through training, recruitment, and retention strategies.

3. Public Health Interventions:

- Implementing public health interventions such as vaccination campaigns, disease surveillance systems, and health education programs to prevent the spread of infectious diseases.

4. Collaboration and Coordination:

- Facilitating multi-sectoral collaboration between government agencies, healthcare providers, community organizations, and international partners to ensure a coordinated response.

5. Communication and Information Sharing:

- Establishing clear communication channels to disseminate accurate information, address public concerns, and combat misinformation during health crises.

Strategies for Long-Term Management in Health Crisis:

1. Adaptive Governance:

- Implementing flexible governance structures that can adapt to changing circumstances and emerging threats.

- Engaging stakeholders in decision-making processes to foster transparency and accountability.

2. Continuous Learning and Improvement:

- Conducting post-event evaluations to identify strengths, weaknesses, and areas for improvement in the response effort.

- Incorporating lessons learned into future planning and management strategies to enhance resilience.

3. Innovation and Technology:

- Harnessing innovative technologies such as telemedicine, digital health platforms, and artificial intelligence to improve healthcare delivery and response capabilities.

4. Community Engagement and Empowerment:

- Engaging communities in the planning, implementation, and evaluation of health crisis response efforts.

- Empowering communities with the knowledge, resources, and skills to effectively participate in disease prevention and control measures.

5. Sustainable Financing:

- Ensuring sustainable financing mechanisms for health emergency preparedness and response activities through government funding, public-private partnerships, and international support.

Conclusion:

Long-term planning and management are essential components of effective health crisis response and recovery efforts. By investing in preparedness, building capacity, fostering collaboration, and adopting innovative strategies, healthcare systems and communities can better mitigate the impact of future health crises and build resilience for the challenges ahead.

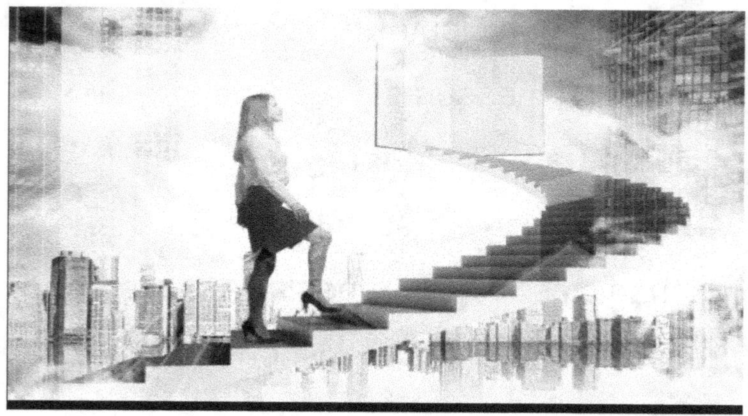

Follow Up Appointments

Introduction:

In times of health crises, such as pandemics or widespread emergencies, managing follow-up appointments becomes crucial for maintaining continuity of care and ensuring optimal health outcomes. This comprehensive guide aims to provide insights and strategies for navigating follow-up appointments during such challenging times, emphasizing the importance of proactive communication, utilizing telemedicine services, and prioritizing essential healthcare needs.

1. Understanding the Importance of Follow-Up Appointments:

- Follow-up appointments play a critical role in monitoring health conditions, adjusting treatment plans, and addressing any emerging issues.

- They are essential for chronic disease management, post-operative care, medication monitoring, and preventive health screenings.

- Skipping or delaying follow-up appointments can lead to worsening health conditions, medication mismanagement, and increased healthcare costs.

2. Proactive Communication with Healthcare Providers:

- Stay informed about any changes in healthcare policies, clinic hours, or appointment protocols during a health crisis.

- Maintain open communication with your healthcare provider or clinic to inquire about the status of your follow-up appointments and any alternative arrangements.

- Discuss any concerns or symptoms you may be experiencing, even if your appointment is postponed, to determine if interim measures or telemedicine consultations are necessary.

3. Utilizing Telemedicine Services:

- Telemedicine offers a convenient and safe alternative to in-person appointments during a health crisis.

- Explore telehealth options provided by your healthcare provider or clinic, including video consultations, phone appointments, and secure messaging platforms.

- Prepare for telemedicine appointments by ensuring a reliable internet connection, familiarizing yourself with the technology platform, and gathering relevant medical information beforehand.

4. Prioritizing Essential Healthcare Needs:

- During a health crisis, healthcare resources may be limited, leading to prioritization of essential services and urgent care.

- Work closely with your healthcare provider to prioritize follow-up appointments based on the urgency of your health condition, medical history, and treatment plan.

- Be flexible and understanding of any rescheduling or adjustments to your follow-up appointments, recognizing the healthcare system's efforts to manage unprecedented challenges.

5. Self-Care and Monitoring:

- Take proactive steps to monitor your health condition between follow-up appointments, such as tracking symptoms, vital signs, and medication adherence.

- Engage in self-care practices, including healthy lifestyle habits, stress management techniques, and adherence to prescribed treatment plans.

- Seek immediate medical attention if you experience any worsening symptoms, emergency situations, or concerns that cannot wait until your next follow-up appointment.

Conclusion:

Navigating follow-up appointments during a health crisis requires proactive communication, utilization of telemedicine services, and prioritization of essential healthcare needs. By staying informed, maintaining open communication with healthcare providers, and taking proactive steps to monitor your health, you can ensure continuity of care and optimal health outcomes despite challenging circumstances.

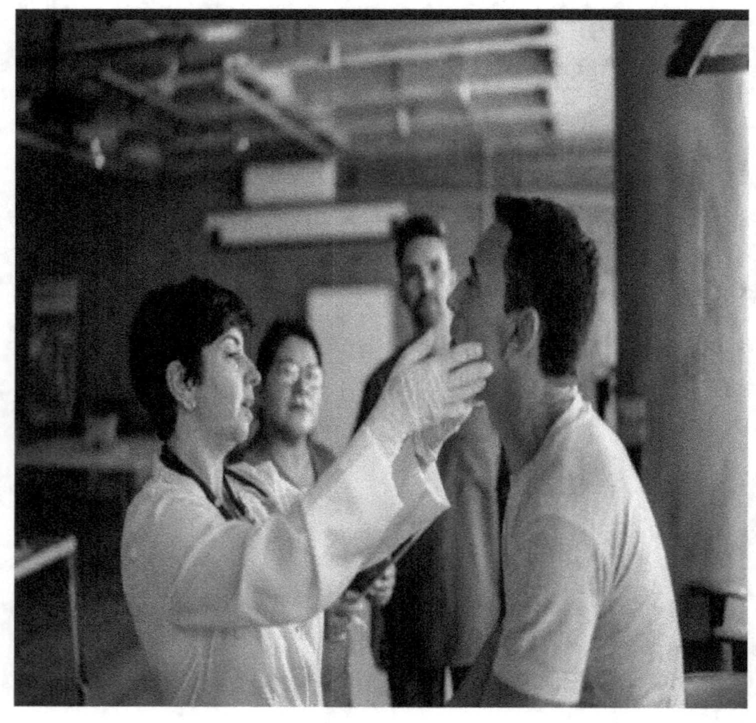

Lifestyle Adjustments

Introduction:

In times of health crises, such as pandemics or widespread diseases, making lifestyle adjustments becomes crucial for maintaining well-being. These adjustments encompass various aspects of life, including physical health, mental well-being, social connections, and daily routines. While navigating through uncertainties and challenges, adopting certain lifestyle changes can help individuals adapt, cope, and even thrive during these challenging times.

1. Prioritize Physical Health:

- **Maintain a Balanced Diet**: Focus on consuming nutritious foods that support your immune system, such as fruits, vegetables, whole grains, lean proteins, and healthy fats.

- **Stay Hydrated**: Drink an adequate amount of water throughout the day to support bodily functions and overall health.

- **Exercise Regularly**: Engage in physical activities suited to your fitness level, whether it's home workouts, yoga, walking, or online exercise classes.

- **Get Sufficient Sleep**: Prioritize quality sleep to boost immunity, improve mood, and enhance overall health.

2. Foster Mental Well-being:

- **Practice Stress Management Techniques**: Incorporate relaxation techniques like deep breathing, meditation, or mindfulness to reduce stress levels.

- **Limit Media Exposure**: Stay informed about the crisis from reliable sources but avoid excessive exposure to distressing news that can contribute to anxiety.

- **Seek Professional Support**: Don't hesitate to reach out to mental health professionals or counselors if you're struggling with anxiety, depression, or other mental health concerns.

- **Maintain Hobbies and Interests**: Engage in activities that bring you joy and fulfillment, whether it's reading, painting, gardening, or playing musical instruments.

3. Cultivate Social Connections:

- **Stay Connected Virtually**: Use technology to stay in touch with friends, family, and loved ones through video calls, social media, or online gaming platforms.

- **Support Others**: Reach out to those who may be isolated or vulnerable, offering assistance, empathy, and companionship.

- **Join Online Communities**: Participate in online forums or groups centered around shared interests, hobbies, or support networks.

- **Practice Empathy and Understanding**: Be compassionate towards others, recognizing that everyone may be experiencing challenges and emotions differently.

4. Adapt Daily Routines:

- **Establish Structure**: Create a daily schedule or routine that provides a sense of normalcy and purpose, including designated work/study hours, meal times, and relaxation periods.

- **Set Realistic Goals**: Break tasks into manageable steps and set achievable goals to maintain motivation and productivity.

- Embrace Flexibility: Be open to adapting your routines and plans as needed to accommodate changes in circumstances or priorities.

- **Incorporate Self-Care Practices**: Dedicate time for self-care activities such as reading, taking a bath, listening to music, or practicing gratitude.

5. Practice Hygiene and Safety Measures:

- **Follow Health Guidelines**: Adhere to recommended hygiene practices, such as frequent handwashing, wearing masks in public spaces, and practicing social distancing.

- **Stay Informed**: Stay updated on the latest health recommendations and guidelines from reputable sources such as the World Health Organization (WHO) or the Centers for Disease Control and Prevention (CDC).

- **Get Vaccinated**: If vaccines are available, prioritize getting vaccinated to protect yourself and others from infectious diseases.

- **Encourage Others**: Advocate for public health measures and encourage others to follow guidelines to collectively reduce the spread of illnesses.

Conclusion:

Navigating through health crises requires resilience, adaptability, and a proactive approach to maintaining well-being. By prioritizing physical health, fostering mental well-being, cultivating social connections, adapting daily routines, and practicing hygiene and safety measures, individuals can effectively navigate challenges and thrive despite the uncertainties. Remember that it's okay to seek support when needed and to prioritize self-care during challenging times. Together, with collective efforts and mindful lifestyle adjustments, we can overcome health crises and emerge stronger as individuals and communities.

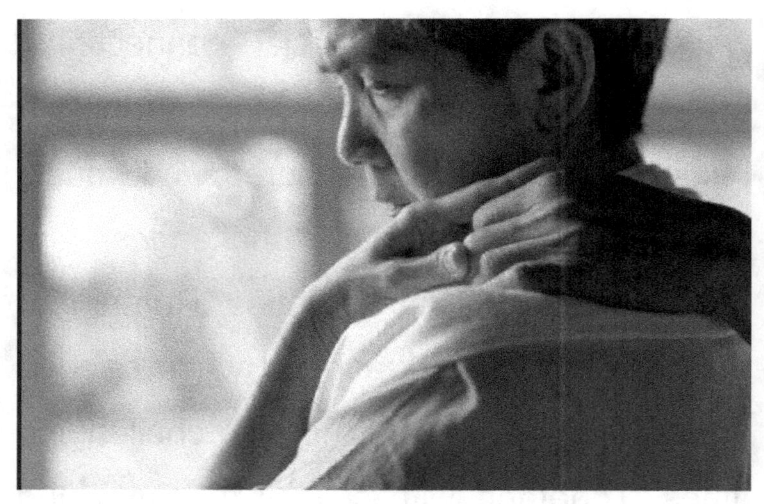

Introduction:

In times of health crises, such as pandemics or natural disasters, the focus often lies on physical health. However, mental health is equally important and can be significantly impacted during such periods. This comprehensive guide aims to highlight the importance of mental health support during health crises and provide strategies and resources to help individuals cope effectively.

Understanding Mental Health Challenges During Health Crises:

1. Increased Stress and Anxiety: Uncertainty, fear of illness, financial concerns, and social isolation can all contribute to heightened stress and anxiety levels.

2. Depression and Isolation: Feelings of loneliness and isolation can exacerbate depression, especially when individuals are separated from their support systems.

3. Trauma and PTSD: Those directly affected by the health crisis, such as frontline workers or survivors of the illness, may experience trauma and develop post-traumatic stress disorder (PTSD).

Strategies for Mental Health Support:

1. Maintain Routine: Establishing and sticking to a daily routine can provide a sense of normalcy and stability during uncertain times.

2. Stay Connected: Utilize technology to stay connected with friends, family, and support groups. Virtual gatherings, video calls, and online communities can offer much-needed social support.

3. Practice Self Care: Prioritize self care activities such as exercise, healthy eating, adequate sleep, and relaxation techniques like meditation or deep breathing exercises.

4. Limit Media Consumption: While it's essential to stay informed, excessive exposure to news and social media can fuel anxiety and distress. Set boundaries on media consumption and take breaks when needed.

5. Seek Professional Help: Don't hesitate to reach out to mental health professionals if you're struggling to cope. Many therapists offer telehealth services, making support accessible from the safety of your home.

Resources for Mental Health Support:

1. Crisis Hotlines: National and local crisis hotlines provide immediate support for individuals in distress. These services are often available 24/7 and offer confidential assistance.

2. Online Therapy Platforms: Platforms like BetterHelp, Talkspace, and 7 Cups offer online therapy sessions with licensed professionals, making mental health support accessible from anywhere.

3. Mental Health Apps: There are numerous apps available for managing stress, anxiety, depression, and other mental health concerns. Examples include Headspace, Calm, and MoodTools.

4. Support Groups: Joining online support groups or forums allows individuals to connect with others facing similar challenges and share experiences and coping strategies.

5. Community Resources: Many community organizations and mental health centers offer support services, including counseling, support groups, and crisis intervention.

Conclusion:

Prioritizing mental health support during health crises is crucial for overall well-being and resilience. By implementing strategies such as maintaining routine, staying connected, and seeking professional help when needed, individuals can better cope with the psychological challenges they may face. Additionally, utilizing resources like crisis hotlines, online therapy platforms, and support groups can provide valuable support and guidance during difficult times. Remember, it's okay to ask for help, and support is available for those who need it.

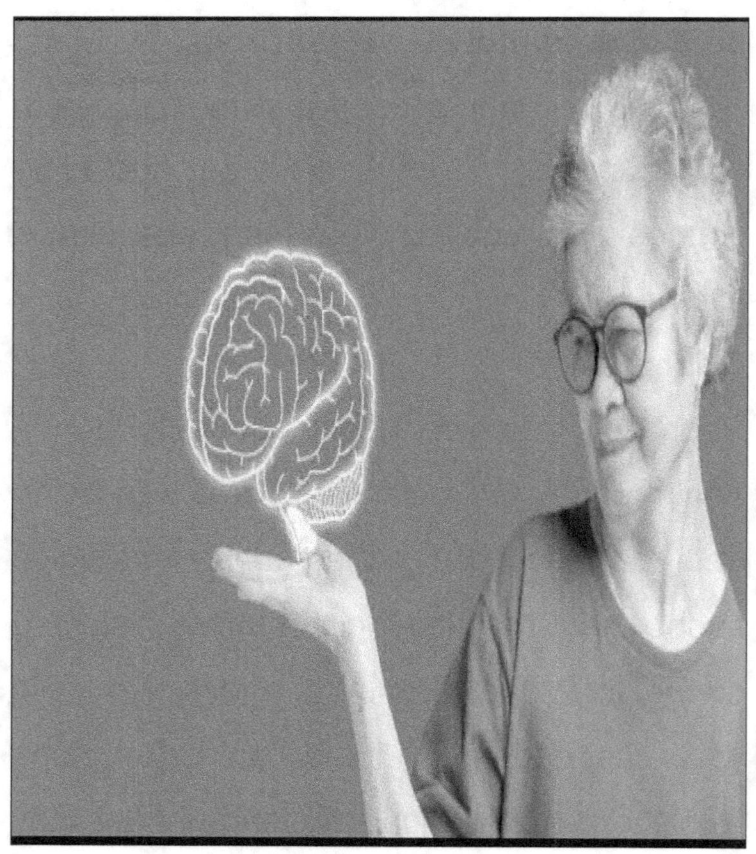

Introduction:

In times of health crises, whether it's a global pandemic, a natural disaster, or a localized outbreak, having access to resources and support systems is crucial for individuals and communities to cope, adapt, and recover. This comprehensive guide aims to explore the various resources and support systems available during health crises and how individuals can utilize them effectively.

1. Understanding Resources:

a. Healthcare Facilities: Hospitals, clinics, and medical centers are primary resources for medical treatment and care during health crises. Understanding their locations, capacities, and services is essential.

b. Medical Supplies: Access to essential medical supplies such as personal protective equipment (PPE), medications, ventilators, and testing kits is vital for healthcare providers and individuals affected by the crisis.

c. Information Channels: Reliable information sources such as government health agencies, WHO, CDC, and local health authorities provide updates, guidelines, and recommendations to navigate the crisis effectively.

d. Financial Assistance: Financial resources, including health insurance coverage, government assistance programs, and charitable organizations, can help individuals manage medical expenses and economic challenges during a health crisis.

e. Mental Health Support: Psychological resources such as counseling services, hotlines, online support groups, and mental health professionals play a crucial role in addressing the emotional impact of a health crisis.

2. Support Systems:

a. Community Networks: Local communities often come together to provide support, solidarity, and assistance during health crises. Community organizations, religious institutions, and volunteer groups offer various forms of aid, including food distribution, shelter, and emotional support.

b. Social Support: Family, friends, and neighbors form an essential support system during challenging times. Building and maintaining social connections can alleviate feelings of isolation and provide practical and emotional support.

c. Peer Support Groups: Connecting with individuals who share similar experiences or conditions can be empowering. Peer support groups offer a platform for sharing experiences, exchanging advice, and fostering a sense of belonging.

d. Telemedicine: Telehealth services enable individuals to access medical care remotely, reducing the burden on healthcare facilities and minimizing exposure to infectious diseases. Virtual consultations, remote monitoring, and teletherapy services are increasingly utilized during health crises.

e. Crisis Intervention Teams: Trained professionals such as crisis counselors, social workers, and mental health experts provide immediate support and intervention during emergencies, helping individuals cope with trauma, grief, and emotional distress.

3. Utilizing Resources and Support Systems:

a. Stay Informed: Regularly seek updates and guidelines from reliable sources to stay informed about the evolving situation and recommended precautions.

b. Access Available Services: Take advantage of healthcare facilities, financial assistance programs, mental health services, and community support initiatives available in your area.

c. Foster Resilience: Cultivate resilience by practicing self-care, maintaining social connections, seeking support when needed, and engaging in coping strategies such as mindfulness, exercise, and hobbies.

d. Advocate for Access: Advocate for equitable access to resources and support systems, particularly for vulnerable populations who may face barriers due to socioeconomic status, language barriers, or discrimination.

e. Support Others: Offer assistance, empathy, and solidarity to those in need within your community, whether it's through volunteering, donating resources, or simply lending a listening ear.

Conclusion:

Navigating a health crisis requires a multifaceted approach that involves leveraging available resources and support systems at individual, community, and societal levels. By understanding, accessing, and utilizing these resources effectively, individuals can mitigate the impact of the crisis and foster resilience in the face of adversity.

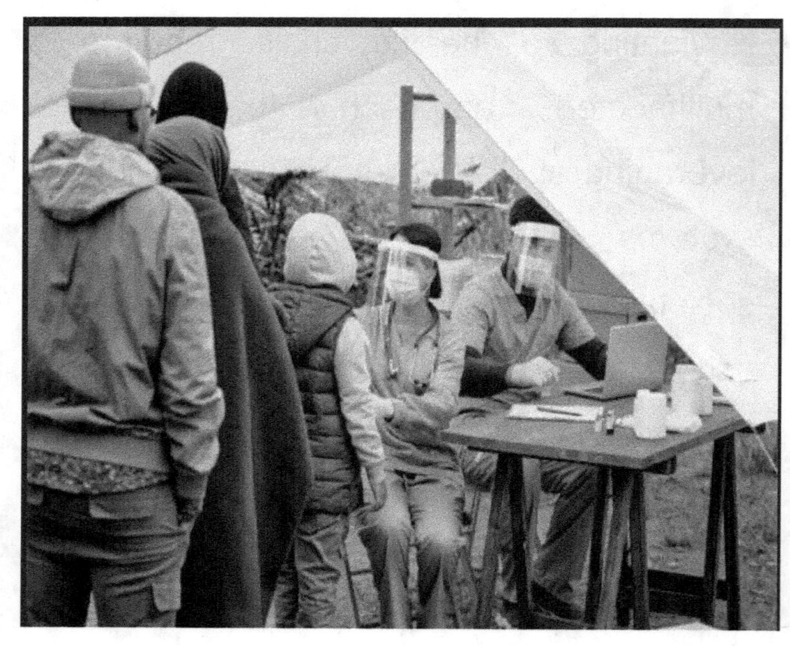

Community Resources

Introduction:

In times of health crises, such as pandemics or natural disasters, communities play a crucial role in providing support, resources, and resilience. This comprehensive guide explores the various community resources available during such crises, highlighting their importance, accessibility, and utilization strategies.

1. Health Services:

   - Local health clinics: Provide medical services, vaccinations, and health education.

- **Mobile clinics**: Reach underserved areas or populations with limited access to healthcare.

- **Telehealth services**: Enable remote consultations and medical advice, reducing the burden on healthcare facilities.

- **Volunteer medical professionals**: Offer their expertise and assistance during crises.

2. **Emergency Response Teams**:

- **Emergency medical services (EMS)**: Respond to medical emergencies and transport patients to hospitals.

- **Disaster response teams**: Provide immediate aid, rescue, and evacuation services during natural disasters or emergencies.

- **Community emergency response teams (CERT)**: Trained volunteers who assist first responders and provide support to affected communities.

3. Mental Health Support:

- **Crisis hotlines**: Offer immediate emotional support and referrals to mental health professionals.

- **Support groups**: Facilitate peer support and coping strategies for individuals facing mental health challenges during crises.

- **Counseling services**: Provide confidential therapy sessions to address trauma, anxiety, and stress related to the crisis.

4. Food Assistance Programs:

- **Food banks**: Distribute food to individuals and families experiencing food insecurity due to economic hardships or 0displacement.

- **Community kitchens**: Offer hot meals and nutritional support to vulnerable populations, including the elderly, children, and homeless individuals.

- **Meal delivery services**: Ensure that homebound or isolated individuals receive nutritious meals during the crisis.

5. Shelter and Housing Support:

- Emergency shelters: Provide temporary housing for individuals displaced by disasters or experiencing homelessness.

- **Housing assistance programs**: Offer financial aid, rental assistance, and supportive services to prevent evictions and homelessness.

- **Temporary housing facilities**: Set up by government agencies or NGOs to accommodate displaced individuals and families during crises.

6. Volunteer Networks:

- Volunteer coordination centers: Mobilize and organize volunteers to assist with various relief efforts, including distribution of supplies, shelter support, and community outreach.

- **Community-based organizations**: Engage local residents in volunteer activities, such as neighborhood clean-ups, wellness checks, and fundraising events.

- Virtual volunteering opportunities: Enable individuals to contribute remotely through online support, fundraising campaigns, and social media outreach.

7. Information and Communication Channels:

- **Public health authorities**: Disseminate accurate and timely information about the crisis, preventive measures, and available resources through websites, social media, and press releases.

- **Community newsletters**: Share updates, resources, and emergency contact information with residents to foster community resilience and preparedness.

- **Community networks**: Utilize radio stations, community bulletin boards, and neighborhood associations to relay important messages and facilitate communication among residents.

Conclusion:

Community resources play a pivotal role in mitigating the impact of health crises by providing essential services, support, and solidarity to affected individuals and families. By harnessing the collective strength and resilience of communities, we can effectively navigate through crises and emerge stronger together.

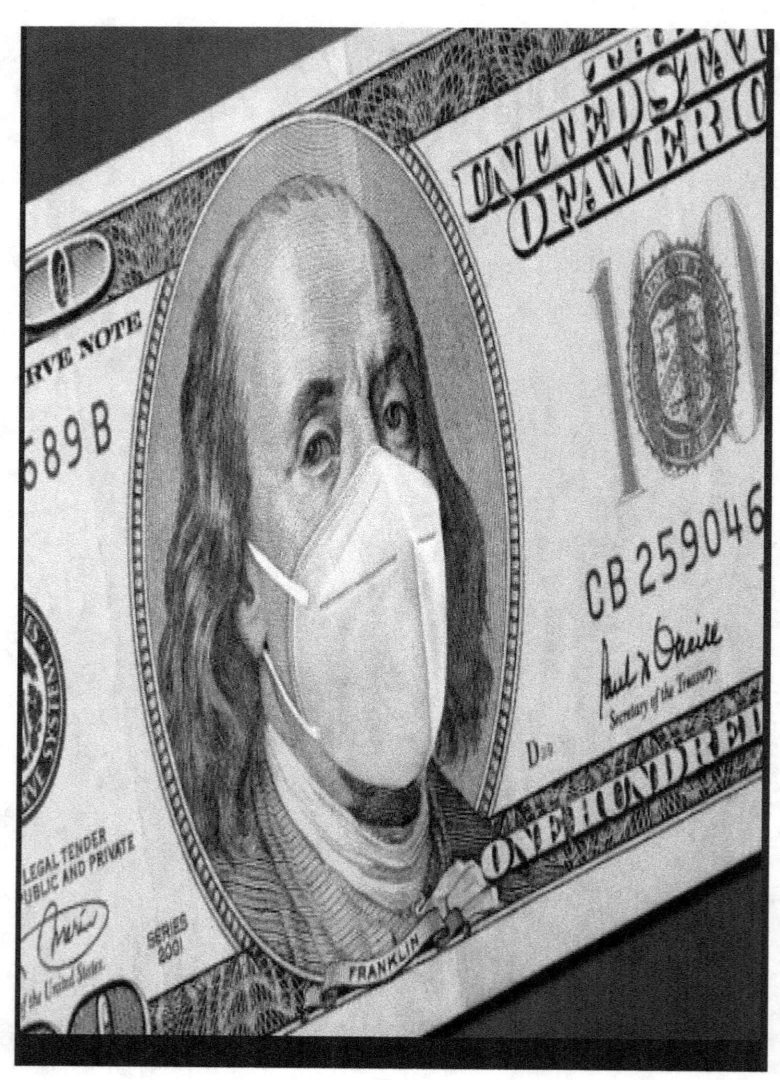

Support Groups

Introduction:

In times of health crises, individuals often find themselves grappling with a myriad of emotions, uncertainties, and challenges. Support groups emerge as invaluable resources providing a sense of community, understanding, and guidance for those navigating through such difficult times. This comprehensive content delves into the significance, types, benefits, and strategies for engaging with support groups during health crises.

Understanding Support Groups:

Support groups are gatherings of individuals who share similar experiences, challenges, or conditions, coming together to offer mutual support, empathy, and encouragement. These groups can take various forms, including in-person meetings, online forums, telephone conferences, or even virtual reality platforms. They cater to a wide range of health crises, such as chronic illnesses, mental health disorders, addiction recovery, grief and loss, and caregiving responsibilities, among others.

Types of Support Groups:

1. **Condition-Specific Groups**: These focus on particular health conditions such as cancer, diabetes, HIV/AIDS, Alzheimer's disease, or rare diseases. Participants share insights, coping strategies, and

medical information specific to their condition.

2. Mental Health Support Groups: These address mental health challenges like depression, anxiety, bipolar disorder, schizophrenia, or PTSD. They provide a safe space for individuals to express themselves, receive validation, and access resources for treatment and management.

3. Caregiver Support Groups: Caregivers of individuals with chronic illnesses, disabilities, or aging-related issues gather to share experiences, practical tips, and emotional support while navigating the demands of caregiving.

4. Bereavement Support Groups: These assist individuals coping with the loss of a loved one, offering compassion, validation of grief, and guidance on the grieving process.

5. Online Communities: Virtual support groups offer accessibility and anonymity, allowing individuals to connect with others facing similar challenges regardless of geographical constraints.

Benefits of Support Groups:

1. Emotional Support: Participants find solace in knowing they are not alone in their struggles and can freely express their feelings without fear of judgment.

2. Information Sharing: Members exchange valuable insights, resources, and practical tips for managing symptoms, treatment options, and navigating the healthcare system.

3. Sense of Belonging: Joining a support group fosters a sense of belonging and camaraderie, reducing feelings of isolation and alienation.

4. Empowerment: Through shared experiences and collective wisdom, individuals feel empowered to take control of their health journey and make informed decisions.

5. Coping Skills Development: Participants learn effective coping mechanisms, resilience strategies, and self-care practices from peers who have faced similar challenges.

6. Improved Mental Health: Regular participation in support groups correlates with reduced feelings of anxiety, depression, and stress, promoting overall psychological well-being.

7. Enhanced Quality of Life: By fostering social connections and emotional resilience, support groups contribute to a higher quality of life despite health crises.

Strategies for Engaging with Support Groups:

1. Research and Select Wisely: Explore different support group options to find one that aligns with your needs, preferences, and goals.

2. Attend Meetings Regularly: Consistent participation fosters trust, rapport, and deeper connections with other members.

3. Actively Participate: Share your experiences, ask questions, offer support to others, and contribute constructively to group discussions.

4. Respect Confidentiality: Maintain confidentiality regarding sensitive information shared within the group to uphold trust and confidentiality.

5. Seek Professional Support When Needed: While support groups offer valuable peer support, they are not substitutes for professional medical or mental health treatment. Seek professional help when necessary.

Conclusion:

In the midst of health crises, support groups serve as lifelines, offering empathy, understanding, and practical guidance to individuals navigating challenging circumstances. By fostering connections, sharing experiences, and offering mutual support, these groups play a crucial role in promoting resilience, empowerment, and improved quality of life amidst adversity. Embracing the collective strength of support groups can empower individuals to navigate their health journey with courage, hope, and resilience.

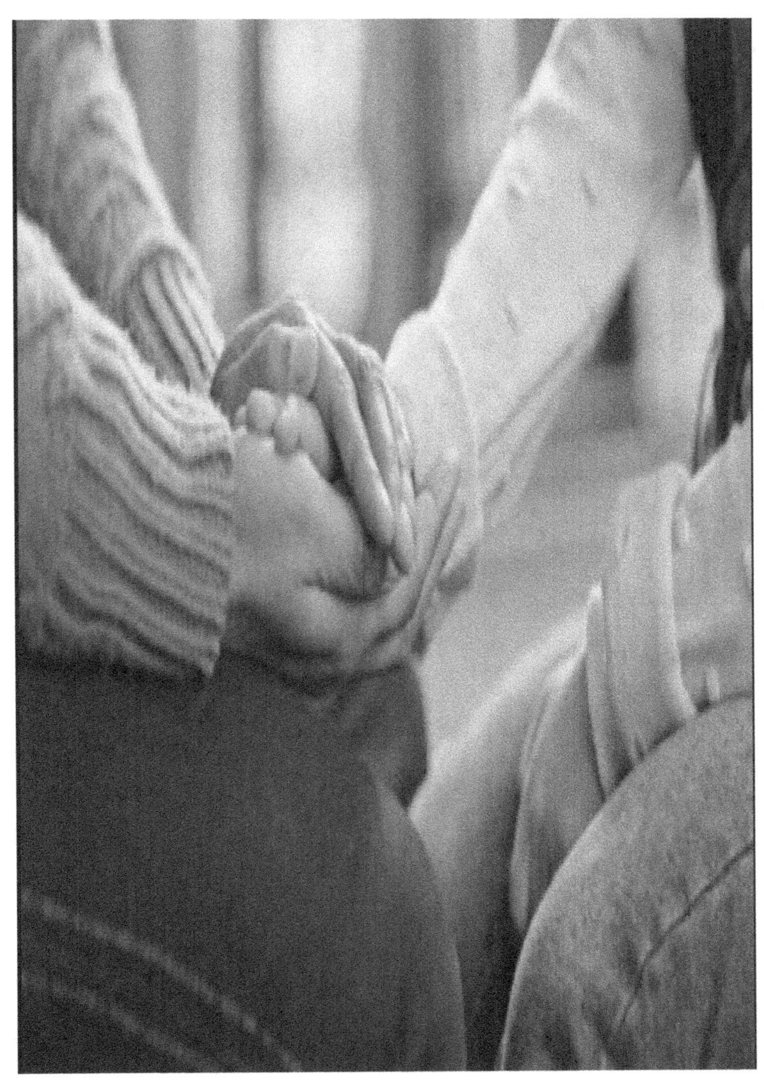

Financial Assistance Options

During times of health crisis, financial assistance can be a lifeline for individuals and families facing medical expenses. Here's a comprehensive overview of various financial assistance options available:

1. Health Insurance Coverage:

- Check your health insurance policy for coverage details regarding medical treatments, hospital stays, and prescription medications.

- Understand your deductible, co-pays, and out-of-pocket maximums to estimate your potential expenses.

- Contact your insurance provider to inquire about any special provisions or coverage extensions during health crises.

2. Government Assistance Programs:

- **Medicaid**: Provides health coverage to low-income individuals and families. Eligibility criteria vary by state.

- **Medicare**: Offers health insurance to people aged 65 and older, as well as certain younger individuals with disabilities.

- **Affordable Care Act (ACA)**: Provides access to affordable health insurance plans through state or federal health insurance marketplaces.

- **Supplemental Security Income (SSI)**: Offers financial assistance to elderly, blind, or disabled individuals with limited income and resources.

3. Hospital Financial Assistance Programs:

- Many hospitals offer financial assistance programs to help patients cover medical bills. These programs often consider factors such as income, household size, and medical expenses.

- Contact the hospital's billing department to inquire about available assistance programs and the application process.

4. Nonprofit Organizations and Charities:

- Various nonprofit organizations and charities provide financial assistance to individuals facing medical crisis.

- Examples include the American Cancer Society, the Leukemia & Lymphoma Society, and the National Organization for Rare Disorders.

5. Prescription Assistance Programs:

- Pharmaceutical companies and nonprofit organizations offer prescription assistance programs to help individuals afford necessary medications.

- These programs may provide discounts, coupons, or free medication to eligible individuals.

6. Crowdfunding and Fundraising:

- Online crowdfunding platforms such as GoFundMe, Kickstarter, and Indiegogo allow individuals to raise funds for medical expenses.

- Share your story with friends, family, and the online community to gather support and financial assistance.

7. Legal Aid and Advocacy Services:

- Seek assistance from legal aid organizations or advocacy groups specializing in healthcare rights and financial assistance.

- These organizations can provide guidance on navigating insurance claims, disputing denied coverage, and accessing available assistance programs.

8. Community Resources:

- Local government agencies, religious organizations, and community centers may offer financial assistance, food assistance, or other support services during health crises.

- Explore community resources and social services available in your area.

9. Negotiation and Payment Plans:

- Contact medical providers and negotiate payment plans or discounts for your medical bills.

- Many healthcare facilities are willing to work with patients to establish manageable payment arrangements.

10. Financial Counseling Services:

- Seek assistance from financial counselors or advisors who specialize in healthcare finance.

- These professionals can help you understand your financial options, create a budget, and navigate the complexities of medical billing.

Remember to thoroughly research and explore all available options for financial assistance during a health crisis. Don't hesitate to reach out to relevant organizations and professionals for guidance and support.

CHAPTER 3 : Review and Reflection

Introduction:

In the face of health crises, whether it be pandemics, natural disasters, or other emergencies, the importance of review and reflection cannot be overstated. These processes serve as crucial tools for assessing response strategies, identifying strengths and weaknesses, and ultimately improving preparedness for future crises. In this comprehensive content, we delve into the significance of review and reflection in health crises, exploring their roles, methodologies, and outcomes.

Understanding Review and Reflection:

Review involves a systematic examination of actions taken during a health crisis, focusing on what was done, how it was done, and why. It aims to assess the effectiveness of response measures, adherence to protocols, and allocation of resources. Reflection, on the other hand, delves deeper into the experiences, emotions, and personal insights gained from the crisis response. It encourages individuals and organizations to contemplate not only what happened but also how they felt, what they learned, and how they can grow from the experience.

Importance of Review and Reflection:

1. Learning from Experience: Review and reflection provide opportunities to learn from both successes and failures encountered during a health crisis. By analyzing past actions and outcomes, stakeholders can identify areas for improvement and implement necessary changes.

2. Enhancing Preparedness: Through review and reflection, healthcare systems and emergency responders can identify gaps in preparedness and response protocols. This allows for adjustments to be made to policies, procedures, and resource allocation, ultimately strengthening readiness for future crises.

3. Building Resilience: By engaging in reflective practices, individuals and organizations develop resilience in the face of adversity. Reflecting on challenges faced and lessons learned fosters adaptability, innovation, and the ability to effectively navigate future crises.

4. Fostering Collaboration: Review and reflection facilitate open dialogue and collaboration among stakeholders involved in crisis response. By sharing experiences, insights, and recommendations, interdisciplinary teams can work together to develop more coordinated and effective response strategies.

Methodologies for Review and Reflection:

1. After-Action Reviews (AARs): AARs involve structured discussions or evaluations conducted after the conclusion of a crisis response. They typically assess what worked well, what did not, and what can be improved, with the goal of capturing lessons learned and identifying areas for enhancement.

2. Peer Reviews: Peer reviews involve the exchange of feedback and insights among colleagues or organizations involved in crisis response. This collaborative approach encourages constructive criticism, shared learning, and the exchange of best practices.

3. Surveys and Interviews: Surveys and interviews can be used to gather feedback from individuals directly involved in crisis response, including healthcare workers, emergency responders, and community members. These methods provide valuable qualitative data on experiences, challenges, and recommendations for improvement.

4. Tabletop Exercises: Tabletop exercises simulate crisis scenarios in a controlled

environment, allowing stakeholders to test response plans, protocols, and communication strategies. These exercises often incorporate elements of review and reflection, providing opportunities for participants to identify strengths and weaknesses in their response efforts.

Outcomes and Implementation:

The outcomes of review and reflection in health crises can vary depending on the context, scale, and severity of the crisis. However, common outcomes include:

- Identification of strengths and weaknesses in crisis response efforts.

- Development of actionable recommendations for improving preparedness and response.

- Enhanced communication and collaboration among stakeholders.

- Increased resilience and adaptability in the face of future crises.

To effectively implement review and reflection processes, it is essential to:

- Establish clear objectives and methodologies for conducting reviews.

- Ensure the participation and engagement of all relevant stakeholders.

- Allocate resources and support for implementing recommendations arising from review and reflection.

- Integrate review and reflection into ongoing preparedness and training efforts.

Conclusion:

Review and reflection are indispensable components of effective crisis management in the realm of public health. By systematically evaluating past actions, learning from experiences, and fostering a culture of continuous improvement, stakeholders can enhance preparedness, build resilience, and mitigate the impact of future health crises. Embracing review and reflection as integral components of crisis response efforts is essential for safeguarding public health and well-being in an ever-changing world.

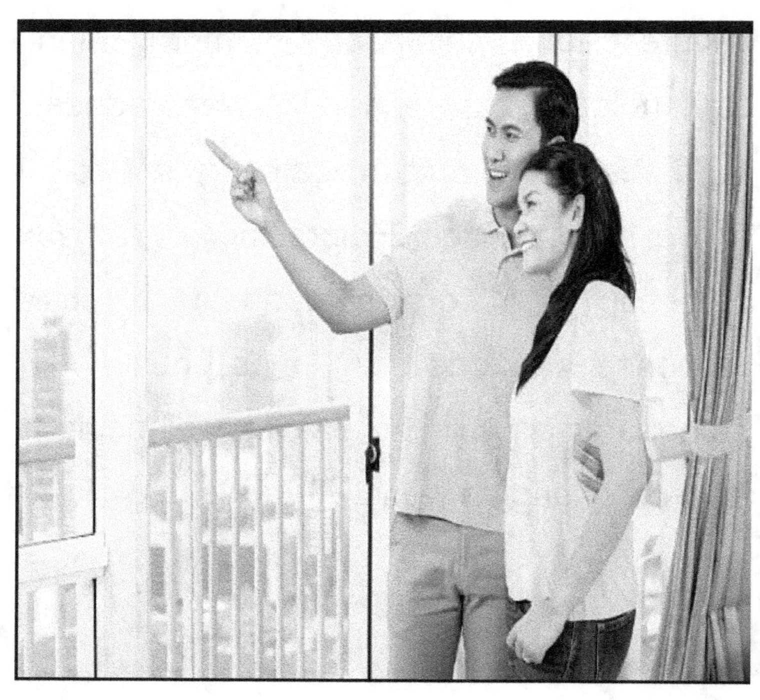

Learning from the Experience

Introduction:

Health crises, whether global pandemics or local outbreaks, present significant challenges to individuals, communities, and healthcare systems worldwide. However, amidst the adversity, these crises offer invaluable opportunities for learning and growth. By reflecting on our experiences, identifying lessons learned, and implementing effective strategies, we can better prepare for and respond to future health emergencies. This comprehensive content explores the key aspects of learning from experience in health crises, highlighting the importance of resilience, adaptability, and collaboration.

1. Resilience in the Face of Adversity:

- Define resilience and its importance in navigating health crises.

- Discuss how individuals and communities can cultivate resilience through coping mechanisms, social support, and adaptive behaviors.

- Share real-life examples of resilience during past health crises, emphasizing the power of human spirit and perseverance.

2. Adaptability: Key to Effective Response:

- Explore the concept of adaptability and its relevance in the context of health emergencies.

- Examine how healthcare systems, organizations, and individuals can adapt their strategies and protocols to changing circumstances.

- Highlight successful examples of adaptability in healthcare delivery, resource management, and public health interventions during previous health crises.

3. Learning from Mistakes and Successes:

- Encourage a culture of reflection and continuous improvement by acknowledging both mistakes and successes in past responses to health crises.

- Analyze common errors and shortcomings in previous crisis management efforts, such as delays in response, misinformation, and inadequate resource allocation.

- Identify best practices and success stories from past experiences, including effective communication strategies, rapid vaccine development, and community engagement initiatives.

4. Collaboration and Coordination:

- Emphasize the importance of collaboration among healthcare professionals, government agencies, NGOs, and the public in responding to health crises.

- Discuss challenges and opportunities for enhancing collaboration across sectors and jurisdictions, including information sharing, resource mobilization, and decision-making processes.

- Showcase examples of successful partnerships and coordinated efforts that have strengthened responses to health emergencies, fostering resilience and solidarity.

5. Building a More Resilient Future:

- Outline actionable steps for individuals, communities, and policymakers to apply lessons learned from past health crises to improve preparedness and response.

- Advocate for investments in public health infrastructure, surveillance systems, and research capabilities to mitigate future risks and vulnerabilities.

- Empower individuals and communities to take proactive measures to protect their health and support each other during times of crisis, fostering a culture of collective resilience and solidarity.

Conclusion:

Learning from experience is essential for building resilience and adapting to the challenges posed by health crises. By reflecting on past responses, identifying lessons learned, and implementing effective strategies, we can better prepare for and respond to future emergencies. Through collaboration, innovation, and a commitment to continuous improvement, we can build a more resilient future where health crises are met with strength, solidarity, and compassion.

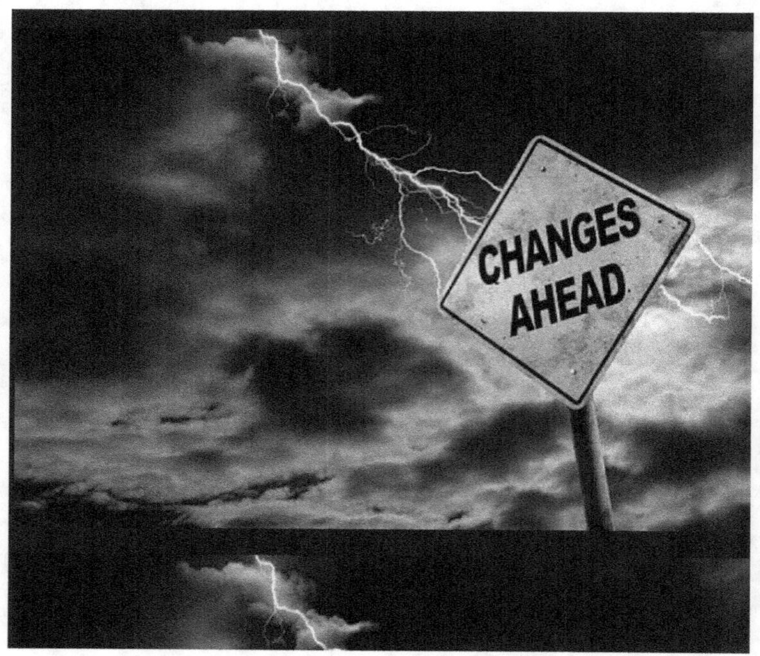

Updating Emergency Plans

Introduction:

In times of health crises such as pandemics or natural disasters, having robust emergency plans in place is crucial for healthcare facilities, organizations, and communities. However, as circumstances evolve and new challenges arise, it's essential to regularly update these plans to ensure they remain effective and responsive to the current situation. This comprehensive guide explores the importance of updating emergency plans in health crises and provides a step-by-step approach to ensure readiness and resilience.

Why Update Emergency Plans in a Health Crisis?

1. Adaptability: Health crises are dynamic and can evolve rapidly, requiring adjustments in response strategies.

2. New Threats: Emerging pathogens or changing environmental factors may present new challenges that necessitate updates to existing plans.

3. Lessons Learned: Evaluating past responses helps identify strengths and weaknesses, enabling improvements for future emergencies.

4. Regulatory Compliance: Compliance with changing regulations and standards requires periodic review and updates of emergency plans.

5. Stakeholder Involvement: Engaging relevant stakeholders ensures inclusivity and enhances the effectiveness of emergency plans.

Steps to Update Emergency Plans:

1. Assessment:

- **Review Current Plan**: Evaluate the existing emergency plan to identify areas for improvement.

- **Risk Assessment**: Identify potential risks and vulnerabilities specific to the current health crisis.

- **Resource Inventory**: Assess available resources, including personnel, equipment, and supplies.

2. Stakeholder Engagement:

- Collaborate with healthcare professionals, local authorities, community leaders, and relevant organizations.

- Seek input from frontline workers and other stakeholders who have firsthand experience during emergencies.

3. Plan Revision:

- Incorporate Lessons Learned: Integrate insights from past emergencies to enhance response strategies.

- **Scenario Planning**: Develop contingency plans for various scenarios based on the evolving nature of the health crisis.

- **Communication Plan**: Establish clear communication protocols to ensure timely dissemination of information to all stakeholders.

4. Training and Drills:

- **Conduct Training Sessions**: Provide regular training to staff members on updated emergency protocols and procedures.

- **Simulation Exercises**: Organize drills and simulations to test the effectiveness of the updated emergency plans in real-life scenarios.

- **Evaluate and Adjust**: Gather feedback from participants and use it to refine the emergency plans further.

5. Resource Allocation:

- Ensure Adequate Resources: Allocate necessary resources such as personal protective equipment (PPE), medical supplies, and staffing based on updated plans.

- Establish Redundancies: Identify backup systems and resources to mitigate the impact of potential shortages or failures.

6. Continuous Monitoring and Evaluation:

- Monitor Key Indicators: Track relevant metrics and indicators to assess the effectiveness of the updated emergency plans.

- **Regular Review**: Schedule periodic reviews to ensure that emergency plans remain aligned with the current situation and evolving needs.

- **Feedback Mechanism**: Establish a mechanism for stakeholders to provide feedback and suggestions for further improvements.

Conclusion:

Updating emergency plans in health crises is an ongoing process that requires proactive assessment, collaboration, and adaptation. By following the steps outlined in this guide, healthcare facilities, organizations, and communities can enhance their readiness and resilience to effectively respond to the challenges posed by evolving health crises. Continuous monitoring, evaluation, and stakeholder engagement are essential to maintaining effective emergency preparedness and ensuring the safety and well-being of individuals and communities.

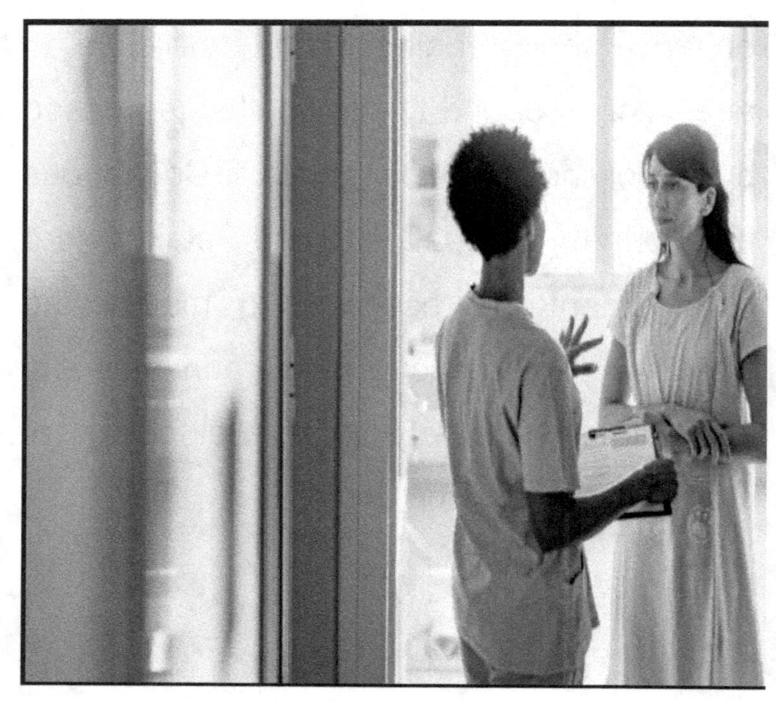

CHAPTER 4 : Building Resilience

Introduction:

In times of health crises, such as pandemics or natural disasters, building resilience becomes paramount for individuals and communities. Resilience refers to the ability to adapt and bounce back from adversity, maintaining mental and emotional well-being despite challenges. This comprehensive guide explores strategies for cultivating resilience in the face of health crises.

Understanding Resilience:

Resilience is not a fixed trait but a dynamic process that can be developed and strengthened over time. It involves various factors, including coping skills, social support, optimism, and self-efficacy. Individuals and communities can proactively work on enhancing these factors to better navigate health crises.

Strategies for Building Resilience:

1. **Cultivate Self-Awareness**: Recognize your emotions, thoughts, and reactions to stress. Practice mindfulness and self-reflection to understand how you cope with challenges and identify areas for improvement.

2. **Foster Social Connections**: Build and maintain strong relationships with family, friends, and community members. Social support networks provide a sense of belonging, emotional support, and practical assistance during difficult times.

3. Develop Coping Skills: Learn effective coping strategies to manage stress and adversity. This may include problem-solving skills, relaxation techniques, positive self-talk, and seeking professional support when needed.

4. Maintain a Healthy Lifestyle: Prioritize self-care activities such as regular exercise, healthy eating, adequate sleep, and relaxation practices. A healthy lifestyle strengthens physical and mental resilience, enabling better coping with health crises.

5. Cultivate Optimism and Adaptability: Foster a positive outlook and belief in your ability to overcome challenges. Embrace change and uncertainty as opportunities for growth and learning. Develop flexible thinking and adaptability to navigate unpredictable situations.

6. Seek Meaning and Purpose: Find meaning in adversity by identifying personal values, goals, and sources of meaning. Engage in activities that bring a sense of purpose and fulfillment, such as helping others, pursuing hobbies, or contributing to community resilience efforts.

7. Build Resilient Communities: Collaborate with neighbors, local organizations, and authorities to create resilient communities. Establish emergency preparedness plans, support systems, and resources to respond effectively to health crises as a collective.

8. Promote Mental Health Awareness: Reduce stigma around mental health issues and encourage open conversations about emotional well-being. Provide access to mental health resources, support services, and education to empower individuals and communities to prioritize mental health during crises.

Conclusion:

Building resilience in health crises is essential for maintaining well-being and thriving despite adversity. By cultivating self-awareness, fostering social connections, developing coping skills, maintaining a healthy lifestyle, fostering optimism, seeking meaning and purpose, building resilient communities, and promoting mental health awareness, individuals and communities can enhance their ability to adapt and thrive in challenging circumstances. Together, we can overcome health crises and emerge stronger and more resilient than before.

Lj

Strengthening Overall Health

Introduction:

Achieving and maintaining overall health is a multifaceted endeavor that involves various aspects of physical, mental, and emotional well-being. By adopting a holistic approach, individuals can strengthen their overall health and enhance their quality of life. This comprehensive guide outlines key strategies for improving overall health, encompassing lifestyle choices, nutrition, exercise, stress management, sleep hygiene, and more.

1. Lifestyle Choices:

- **Regular Physical Activity**: Engage in moderate to vigorous exercise for at least 150 minutes per week, incorporating cardiovascular, strength training, and flexibility exercises.

- **Healthy Diet**: Consume a balanced diet rich in fruits, vegetables, whole grains, lean proteins, and healthy fats while limiting processed foods, added sugars, and excessive salt intake.

- **Avoidance of Harmful Substances**: Minimize or eliminate tobacco, alcohol, and illicit drug use to reduce the risk of chronic diseases and improve overall well-being.

- **Maintaining a Healthy Weight**: Strive for a healthy weight through a combination of nutritious eating habits and regular physical activity to lower the risk of obesity-related conditions such as diabetes, heart disease, and certain cancers.

2. Nutrition:

- **Portion Control**: Be mindful of portion sizes to prevent overeating and maintain a healthy weight.

- **Hydration**: Drink an adequate amount of water throughout the day to support bodily functions, promote digestion, and maintain hydration.

- **Nutrient-Rich Foods**: Prioritize foods that are nutrient-dense, such as fruits, vegetables, whole grains, lean proteins, and healthy fats, to provide essential vitamins, minerals, and antioxidants.

3. Exercise:

- **Cardiovascular Exercise**: Engage in activities such as walking, running, swimming, cycling, or dancing to improve heart health, increase endurance, and boost mood.

- **Strength Training**: Incorporate resistance training exercises using weights, resistance bands, or body weight to build muscle strength, improve metabolism, and enhance bone density.

- **Flexibility and Balance**: Practice stretching exercises, yoga, or tai chi to enhance flexibility, balance, and coordination, reducing the risk of falls and injuries.

4. Stress Management:

- **Mindfulness and Meditation**: Cultivate mindfulness through meditation, deep breathing exercises, or mindfulness-based practices to reduce stress, promote relaxation, and enhance mental clarity.

- **Time Management**: Prioritize tasks, delegate responsibilities, and set boundaries to manage time effectively and reduce feelings of overwhelm.

- **Healthy Coping Mechanisms**: Develop healthy coping strategies such as journaling, spending time in nature, engaging in hobbies, or seeking support from friends and family to deal with stressors effectively.

5. Sleep Hygiene:

- **Establish a Routine**: Maintain a consistent sleep schedule by going to bed and waking up at the same time each day, even on weekends.

- **Create a Relaxing Environment**: Make your bedroom conducive to sleep by minimizing noise, light, and electronic distractions.

- Practice Relaxation Techniques: Wind down before bedtime with relaxation techniques such as reading, taking a warm bath, or practicing gentle yoga to promote restful sleep.

6. Regular Health Checkups:

- Preventive Screenings: Schedule regular checkups with healthcare providers for preventive screenings, vaccinations, and health assessments to detect and manage any potential health issues early.

- Open Communication: Communicate openly with healthcare providers about any concerns, symptoms, or changes in health to receive appropriate guidance and support.

Conclusion:

By incorporating these strategies into daily life, individuals can strengthen their overall health and well-being, fostering a balanced and sustainable approach to living. Prioritizing healthy lifestyle choices, nutrition, exercise, stress management, sleep hygiene, and regular health checkups can empower individuals to lead vibrant and fulfilling lives. Remember, small changes over time can lead to significant improvements in overall health and vitality.

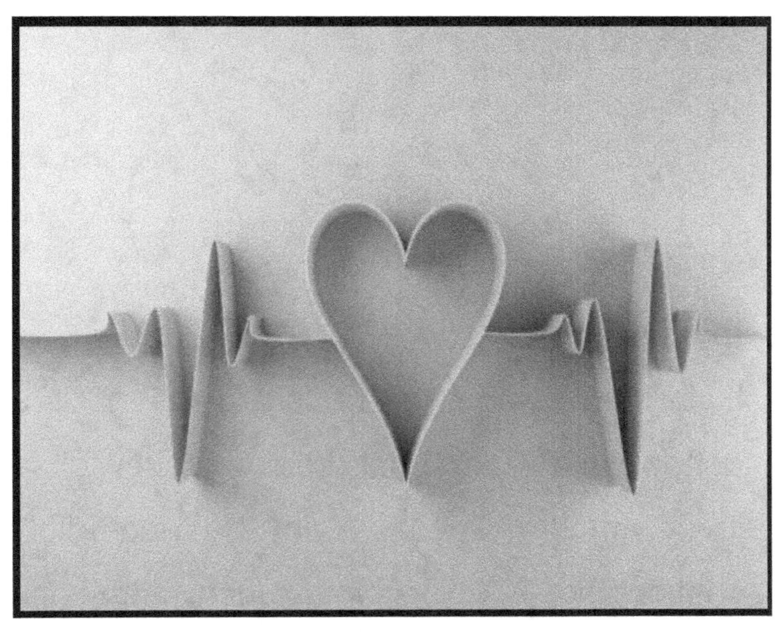

Developing Coping Strategies

Introduction:

Living through a health crisis, whether it's a pandemic, a personal health issue, or a loved one's illness, can be incredibly challenging. Coping with such situations requires resilience, adaptability, and a proactive approach to managing stress and uncertainty. This comprehensive guide explores various coping strategies individuals can employ to navigate health crises effectively.

Understanding Coping:

Coping involves the cognitive and behavioral efforts individuals make to manage stressful situations, emotions, and thoughts. Effective coping strategies can help reduce anxiety, improve emotional well-being, and enhance overall resilience.

Types of Coping Strategies:

1. Emotion-Focused Coping: These strategies focus on managing emotions associated with the crisis. Examples include relaxation techniques, mindfulness meditation, and engaging in activities that bring joy and comfort.

2. Problem-Focused Coping: These strategies involve tackling the root cause of stressors. Examples include seeking information about the health crisis, developing action plans, and problem-solving.

3. Social Support: Connecting with friends, family, or support groups can provide emotional comfort and practical assistance during difficult times. Sharing experiences and feelings with others who understand can alleviate feelings of isolation.

4. Self-Care Practices: Prioritizing self-care is essential for maintaining physical and mental well-being during a health crisis. This includes adequate sleep, nutrition, exercise, and relaxation activities.

5. Cognitive Restructuring: This involves challenging negative thoughts and reframing them in a more positive or realistic light. Techniques such as cognitive-behavioral therapy (CBT) can help individuals develop healthier thinking patterns.

6. Maintaining Routine: Establishing and sticking to a daily routine can provide structure and stability amidst uncertainty. Routine activities can offer a sense of control and normalcy during challenging times.

Developing Coping Strategies:

1. Self-Awareness: Recognize your emotions, thoughts, and physical sensations related to the health crisis. Self-awareness is the first step in developing effective coping strategies.

2. Seek Information: Educate yourself about the health crisis, including its causes, symptoms, and available resources for support and treatment. Understanding the situation can reduce feelings of uncertainty and fear.

3. Identify Support Systems: Reach out to friends, family, healthcare professionals, or support groups for emotional and practical support. Don't hesitate to ask for help when needed.

4. Practice Self Care: Prioritize activities that promote physical and mental well-being, such as exercise, relaxation techniques, hobbies, and spending time in nature.

5. Develop Coping Skills: Experiment with different coping strategies to find what works best for you. Keep a journal to track your experiences and identify patterns of what helps alleviate stress.

6. **Stay Flexible**: Be open to adjusting your coping strategies as the situation evolves. What worked yesterday may not work today, so stay flexible and adaptable in your approach.

Conclusion:

Developing coping strategies during a health crisis is essential for maintaining resilience and well-being. By understanding different coping techniques and implementing them effectively, individuals can navigate challenging times with greater ease and emerge stronger from the experience. Remember, coping is a personal journey, so be patient and compassionate with yourself as you find what works best for you.

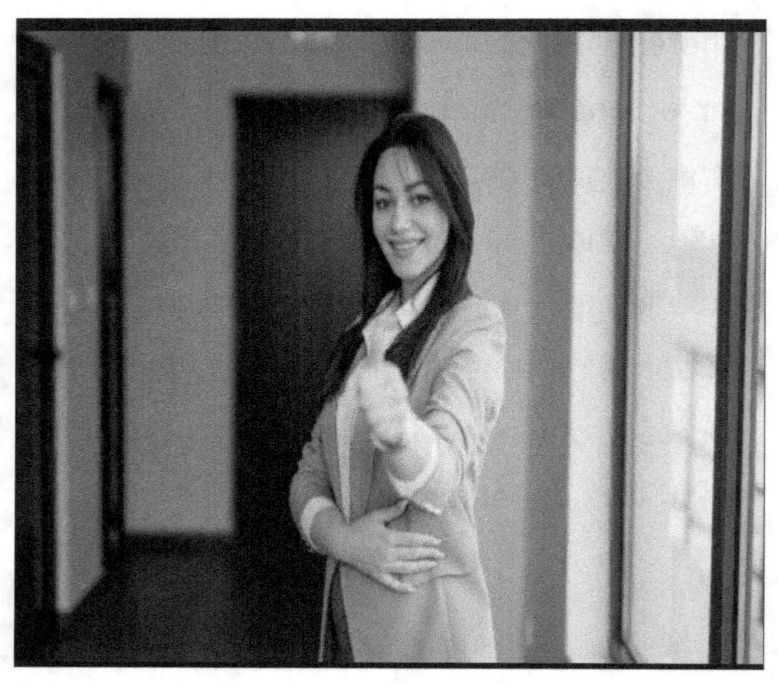

Introduction:

In times of health crises, proactive prevention measures are paramount in safeguarding public health and mitigating the spread of diseases. This comprehensive guide aims to outline various strategies and actions to encourage individuals and communities to adopt preventive measures effectively.

1. Education and Awareness:

- Provide clear, accurate, and accessible information about the health crisis, including its causes, symptoms, transmission methods, and preventive measures.

- Utilize various communication channels such as social media, television, radio, and community outreach programs to disseminate information.

- Address misinformation and myths surrounding the health crisis through factual education campaigns.

2. Promotion of Hygiene Practices:

- Emphasize the importance of frequent handwashing with soap and water for at least 20 seconds.

- Encourage the use of alcohol-based hand sanitizers when handwashing facilities are not available.

- Promote respiratory hygiene, including covering coughs and sneezes with a tissue or elbow, and proper disposal of tissues.

3. Adoption of Social Distancing Measures:

- Advocate for maintaining physical distance from others, avoiding large gatherings, and implementing remote work and online schooling where feasible.

- Encourage the use of face masks or face coverings in public settings, especially where maintaining physical distance is challenging.

4. Support for Vaccination:

- Promote vaccination as a crucial preventive measure against the health crisis, highlighting the safety and efficacy of approved vaccines.

- Address vaccine hesitancy through targeted communication campaigns that address concerns and provide factual information.

5. Encouragement of Healthy Lifestyle Choices:

- Stress the importance of maintaining a healthy lifestyle, including regular exercise, balanced nutrition, adequate sleep, and stress management techniques.

- Provide resources and support for smoking cessation, as smoking can exacerbate the severity of certain health crises.

6. Community Engagement and Empowerment:

- Foster a sense of collective responsibility within communities by encouraging individuals to take ownership of their health and the health of others.

- Facilitate community-led initiatives and partnerships to implement preventive measures tailored to local contexts and needs.

7. Recognition and Reward Systems:

- Implement incentives and recognition programs to acknowledge individuals, businesses, and communities that demonstrate exemplary adherence to preventive measures.

- Highlight success stories and positive outcomes resulting from the adoption of preventive measures to inspire others to follow suit.

8. Continuous Monitoring and Evaluation:

- Establish mechanisms for ongoing monitoring and evaluation of preventive measures to assess their effectiveness and identify areas for improvement.

- Use data driven insights to refine strategies, allocate resources efficiently, and address emerging challenges in real-time.

Conclusion:

Encouraging preventive measures in health crises requires a multi faceted approach that encompasses education, promotion of hygiene practices, social distancing, vaccination support, healthy lifestyle choices, community engagement, recognition systems, and continuous monitoring and evaluation. By empowering individuals and communities to take proactive steps to protect themselves and others, we can effectively combat health crises and promote overall well-being.

CHAPTER 5 : Helping Friends and Family in Crisis

Introduction:

In times of crisis, whether it be a personal tragedy, financial hardship, or health issue, our friends and family often turn to us for support. Being there for loved ones during tough times is not only essential for their well-being but can also strengthen bonds and foster resilience. This comprehensive guide explores various ways to help friends and family in crisis, offering practical tips and strategies for providing meaningful support.

1. Active Listening and Empathy:

- **Listen without judgment**: Allow your loved one to express their thoughts and feelings without interrupting or offering unsolicited advice.

- **Practice empathy**: Try to understand their perspective and validate their emotions by acknowledging their feelings without trying to fix them.

2. Offering Practical Assistance:

- **Identify specific needs**: Ask your loved one how you can best support them and offer practical help such as running errands, cooking meals, or providing transportation.

- **Coordinate support**: Organize a schedule among friends and family members to ensure continuous assistance without overwhelming any single individual.

3. Providing Emotional Support:

- **Be present**: Simply being there for your loved one, whether physically or virtually, can provide immense comfort and reassurance.

- **Express care and concern**: Offer words of encouragement, reassurance, and affection to let them know they are not alone in their struggles.

4. Respecting Boundaries:

- **Respect their autonomy**: While it's essential to offer support, respect your loved one's boundaries and avoid imposing your own agenda or expectations on them.

- **Offer space when needed**: Recognize when your loved one needs time alone or space to process their emotions, and be understanding of their need for solitude.

5. Encouraging Professional Help:

- **Normalize seeking professional support**: Encourage your loved one to seek help from a therapist, counselor, or support group if they are struggling to cope with their crisis.

- **Offer to assist with logistics**: Help them research therapists, schedule appointments, or accompany them to their sessions if needed.

6. Fostering Self-Care:

- **Encourage self-care practices**: Remind your loved one of the importance of self-care activities such as exercise, mindfulness, and hobbies that bring them joy.

- **Lead by example**: Demonstrate self-care behaviors in your own life and encourage your loved one to prioritize their well-being during difficult times.

7. Maintaining Long-Term Support:

- **Continue to check in**: Even after the immediate crisis has passed, continue to check in regularly with your loved one to see how they are doing and offer ongoing support.

- **Be patient and understanding**: Healing from a crisis takes time, so be patient and understanding as your loved one navigates their journey toward recovery.

Conclusion:

Supporting friends and family through crisis ljrequires compassion, empathy, and a willingness to be there for them in their time of need. By actively listening, offering practical assistance, providing emotional support, respecting boundaries, encouraging professional help, fostering self-care, and maintaining long-term support, you can make a meaningful difference in the lives of those you care about during their most challenging moments. Remember, your presence and support can be a source of strength and comfort during their darkest times.

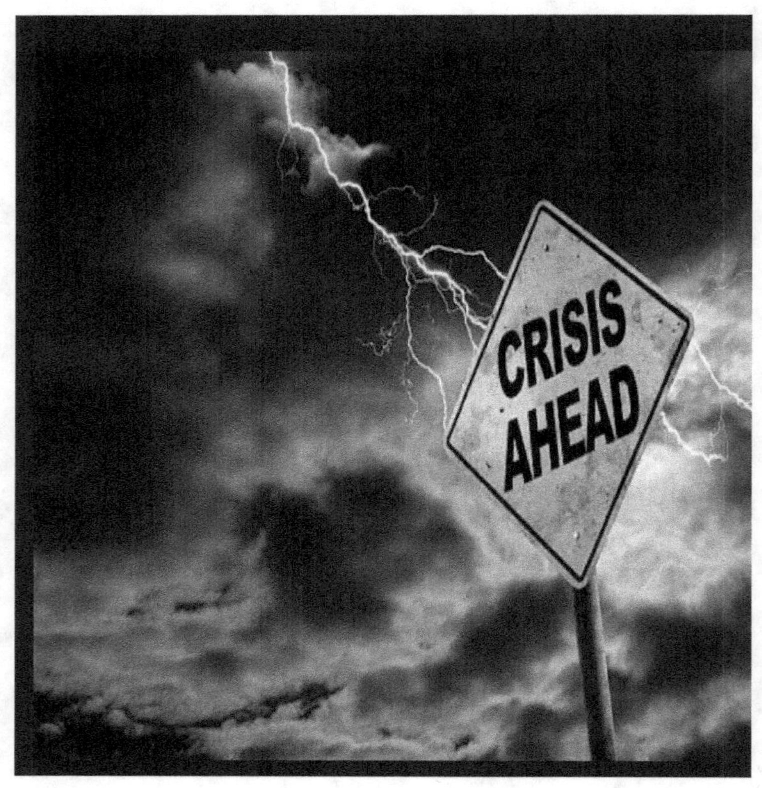

Providing Emotional Support

Introduction:

During health crises, individuals not only face physical challenges but also encounter significant emotional distress. Providing effective emotional support is crucial in helping individuals cope with the uncertainty, fear, and anxiety that accompany such situations. This comprehensive guide aims to outline strategies and techniques for offering emotional support in health crises.

Understanding Emotional Needs:

1. Recognize Emotions: Acknowledge the range of emotions individuals may experience, including fear, anxiety, sadness, anger, and confusion.

2. Empathy: Demonstrate empathy by actively listening, validating feelings, and showing understanding without judgment.

3. Cultural Sensitivity: Be mindful of cultural differences and how they may influence emotional expressions and coping mechanisms.

Building Supportive Relationships:

1. Establish Trust: Create a safe and supportive environment where individuals feel comfortable expressing their emotions openly.

2. Communication: Foster open communication channels to encourage individuals to share their concerns, fears, and needs.

3. Confidentiality: Respect confidentiality and privacy to maintain trust and confidentiality.

Providing Practical Support:

1. Information Sharing: Offer accurate and relevant information about the health crisis, treatment options, and available resources to empower individuals to make informed decisions.

2. Access to Resources: Provide access to support services, such as counseling, support groups, hotlines, and online forums, to help individuals connect with others facing similar challenges.

3. Assistance with Activities of Daily Living: Offer assistance with practical tasks, such as meal preparation, transportation, and household chores, to alleviate stress and burden.

Emotional Support Techniques:

1. Active Listening: Practice active listening by giving full attention, maintaining eye contact, and responding empathetically to verbal and non-verbal cues.

2. Validation: Validate individuals' emotions by acknowledging their feelings as valid and understandable.

3. Encouragement: Offer words of encouragement, reassurance, and optimism to instill hope and resilience.

4. Self Care: Encourage individuals to prioritize self-care activities, such as exercise, relaxation techniques, hobbies, and social connections, to manage stress and maintain emotional well-being.

5. Professional Help: Recognize when individuals may benefit from professional mental health support and encourage them to seek help from qualified professionals, such as therapists, counselors, or psychologists.

Supporting Caregivers:

1. Recognize Caregiver Needs: Acknowledge the emotional challenges and stressors faced by caregivers, including burnout, guilt, and isolation.

2. Respite Care: Offer respite care options to give caregivers a break and time for self-care.

3. Support Groups: Facilitate support groups or peer networks for caregivers to share experiences, strategies, and emotional support.

Conclusion:

Providing emotional support in health crises requires a holistic approach that addresses individuals' emotional needs, fosters supportive relationships, provides practical assistance, and utilizes effective support techniques. By offering compassionate care and understanding, we can help individuals navigate through challenging times with resilience and hope.

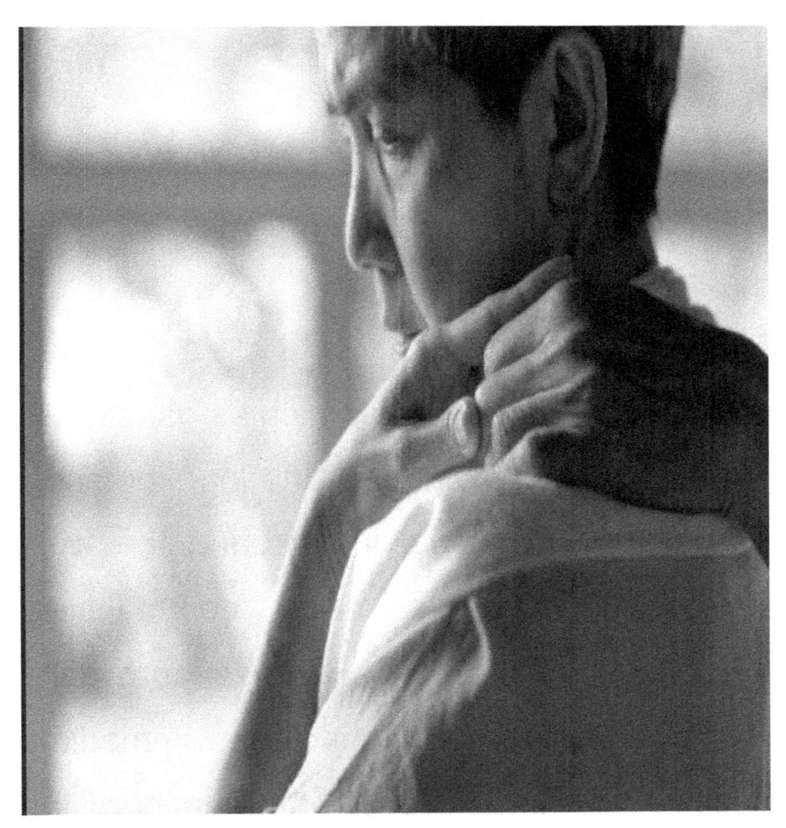

Offering Practical Assistance

Introduction:

In times of health crises, such as pandemics or natural disasters, offering practical assistance is crucial in ensuring the well-being of individuals and communities. Practical assistance involves providing tangible support that addresses immediate needs and helps mitigate the impact of the crisis. This comprehensive guide outlines various ways individuals, organizations, and communities can offer practical assistance during health crises.

1. Assessing Needs:

- Before offering assistance, it's essential to assess the specific needs of the affected individuals and communities.

- Conduct surveys, interviews, or collaborate with local authorities and organizations to identify the most pressing needs, such as food, shelter, medical supplies, or mental health support.

2. Mobilizing Resources:

- Once the needs are identified, mobilize resources to address them effectively.

- This may involve coordinating with government agencies, NGOs, businesses, and volunteers to gather supplies, funds, and manpower.

3. Providing Medical Assistance:

- In health crises, medical assistance is often paramount.

- Set up medical camps, mobile clinics, or telemedicine services to provide basic healthcare services to those in need.

- Distribute essential medical supplies such as masks, sanitizers, medicines, and hygiene kits.

4. Ensuring Access to Food and Water:

- Access to nutritious food and clean water is critical for survival, especially during health emergencies.

- Establish food distribution centers, community kitchens, or food banks to ensure everyone has access to adequate nutrition.

- Provide safe drinking water through filtration systems or distribution of bottled water.

5. Offering Shelter and Protection:

- Many individuals may be displaced or homeless during health crises, requiring immediate shelter and protection.

- Set up temporary shelters in safe locations, equipped with basic amenities such as bedding, sanitation facilities, and security.

- Ensure shelters are accessible to vulnerable populations such as the elderly, children, and people with disabilities.

6. Supporting Mental Health:

- Health crises can take a toll on mental well-being, leading to anxiety, stress, and trauma.

- Provide psychological first aid, counseling services, and support groups to help individuals cope with emotional distress.

- Promote self-care practices and resilience-building activities to strengthen mental health resilience.

7. Promoting Hygiene and Sanitation:

- Hygiene and sanitation are essential for preventing the spread of diseases during health crises.

- Conduct hygiene awareness campaigns, distribute hygiene kits, and provide access to sanitation facilities such as toilets and handwashing stations.

- Promote proper handwashing techniques and respiratory hygiene practices.

8. Facilitating Information and Education:

- Information dissemination is crucial for raising awareness and empowering individuals to protect themselves during health crises.

- Provide accurate and timely information about preventive measures, symptoms, available services, and support resources.

- Offer educational programs, workshops, and training sessions on health and hygiene practices.

9. Engaging Community Participation:

- Engage the community in the planning, implementation, and monitoring of assistance programs.

- Foster partnerships and collaboration between local stakeholders, community leaders, and volunteers to ensure a coordinated response.

- Empower community members to take active roles in assisting their peers and neighbors.

Conclusion:

Offering practical assistance in health crises requires a concerted effort involving various stakeholders, resources, and strategies. By assessing needs, mobilizing resources, and implementing targeted interventions, individuals, organizations, and communities can make a significant difference in alleviating the impact of health emergencies and promoting resilience and recovery. Together, we can build stronger, more resilient communities that are better prepared to face future health challenges.

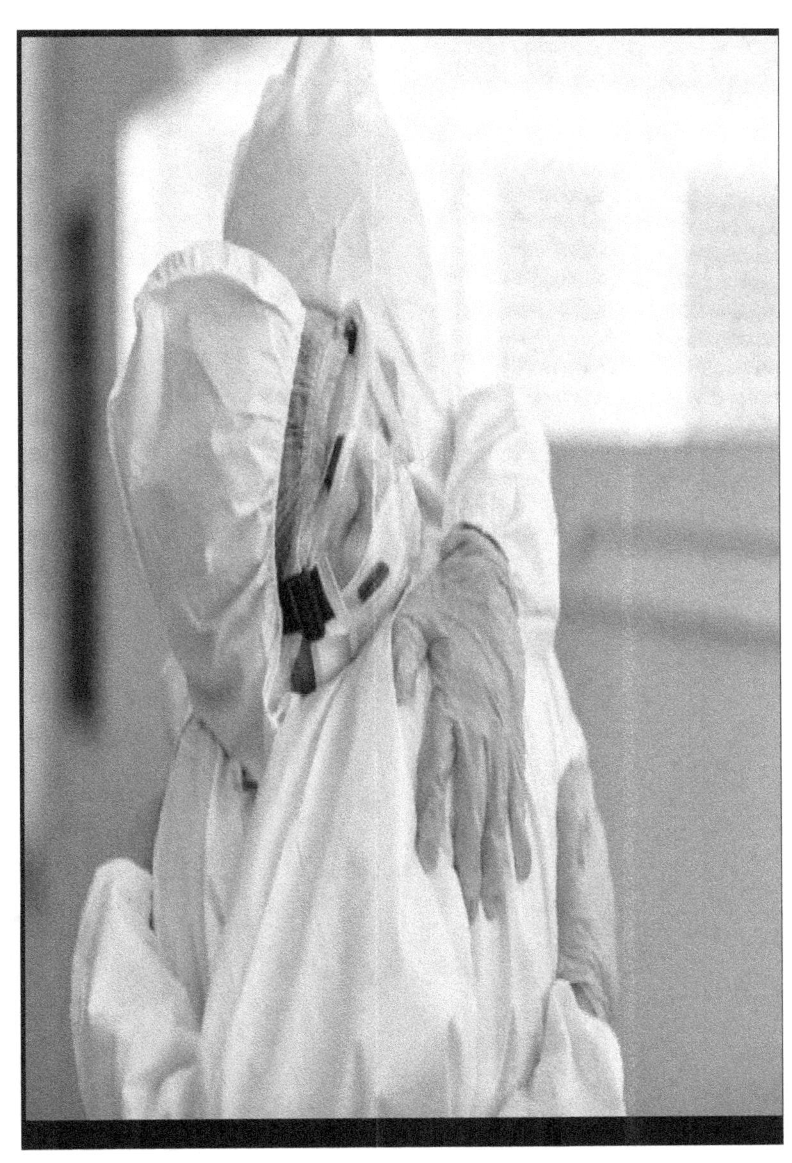

www.ingramcontent.com/pod-product-compliance
Lightning Source LLC
Chambersburg PA
CBHW071222260726
48653CB00042B/1720